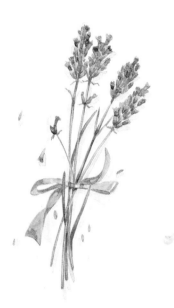

THE ART OF

Aromatherapy

A Guide to Using Essential Oils for Health and Relaxation

PAMELA ALLARDICE

CRESCENT BOOKS

NEW YORK • AVENEL, NEW JERSEY

Contents

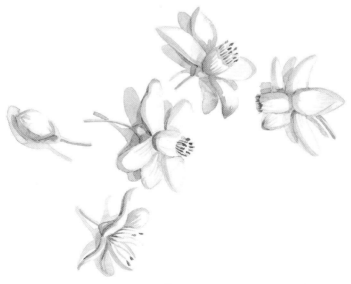

Introduction

Since ancient times essential oils have been thought to benefit the body, mind and emotions. Old manuscripts tell of fragrances from plants as ingredients in charms and ceremonies, as well as in remedies, cosmetics, and food. In the Middle Ages, in particular, monks cultivated herbs and discovered many of their restorative properties. They were among the first to distil precious plant essences, carefully blending them into liqueurs to be administered to patients.

These concentrated pure plant extracts, revered for their fragrance and their therapeautic value, are what we term essential oils. The use of such oils is known as aromatherapy.

Many essential oils are believed to have special properties, ranging from antiseptic to aphrodisiac in effect. Some promote relaxation and a general feeling of balance, others stimulate and rejuvenate. All can encourage a feeling of well-being and can be used to treat or prevent health problems, or simply to create a mood and pamper your senses.

Particular essential oils may be prescribed by an aromatherapist for varying conditions. Chamomile is useful for tension and insomnia; rosemary is good for poor circulation and fatigue; peppermint is a tried and true remedy for indigestion; common sage can benefit muscular problems; and sandalwood has a relaxing and tonifying effect on the nervous system.

There are many ways to experience the benefits of essential oils, which involve either breathing in the enticing aromas or absorbing the diluted oils through the skin. Because essential oils are highly concentrated, it is not usually advisable to apply them directly to your skin or to inject them, unless advised by a skilled therapist.

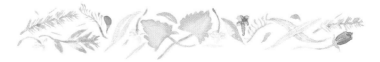

AROMATHERAPY MASSAGE

Essential oils penetrate the skin very quickly to reach the bloodstream and are therefore a marvellous accessory to massage therapy. The concentrated oil should be added to a much greater quantity of oil known as a "carrier" or "base" oil. These should have a neutral odour and be easily absorbed. Light vegetable or nut oils such as almond, apricot kernel, grapeseed, soya, and peach kernel are popular choices.

Do not make up too much massage oil at one time as the fragrance spoils after a short while. A few drops of your selected essential oil in three tablespoons of carrier oil should be sufficient for a massage. Adding wheatgerm oil or vitamin E to your mixture can help to prevent it from turning rancid. Store your massage oil in a corked bottle or a flip-top plastic bottle. The latter is more convenient as it is less likely to spill. Dark glass bottles are best for reducing deterioration of essential oils in any form.

AROMATIC BATHS

An important part of aromatherapy, aromatic baths can be detoxifying, relaxing, or reviving, depending on the oil or oils you choose. They are wonderful just before bed at night, both to help reduce pain or to dispel stress which may keep you awake.

To prepare an aromatherapy bath, simply add two to four drops of your selected oil(s) to a warm bath, stir to ensure the oil is evenly dispersed, and then relax in the scented water. A ten-minute soak should have the desired effect. Variations on aromatic bathing include a sitz or hip bath, or footbaths. Essential oils may also be used in the shower and on compresses to ease muscular aches, sprains and bruises.

INHALANTS OR ROOM FRESHENERS

The various essential oils have different influences on mood. To use them as an inhalant or as a room freshener, try experimenting with the following combinations:

- to stimulate the mind: rosemary, sage, or thyme
- to create a feminine aura: rose, geranium, jasmine
- to complement a celebration, such as a wedding: rose, jasmine
- to clear the mind for psychic healing: lavender, sandalwood, lemongrass
- for a healing atmosphere in a sick-room: rose, bay, thyme
- for meditation: lavender, ylang ylang, jasmine.

Inhalations may be used to relieve headaches and clear the congestion that accompanies colds or sinusitis. To make a simple steam inhalation, add two to four drops of your selected essential oil — eucalyptus, thyme, and tea tree are recommended — to a bowl of very hot water, lean over, tent your head with a towel, and breathe in the vapour for at least three to five minutes.

To disseminate essential oils in a wider environment, clay or ceramic vapourizers are used to heat water with, or near, the oils. Electric vapourizers are also available, as are light bulb rings. These hollow clay rings contain the essential oil and are slipped over light bulbs so that the room is filled with fragrance once a bulb heats up. Simplest of all these methods is the plastic pump spray bottle: just fill with water and selected essential oil, shake and use to mist a room and enliven it with fresh scent.

The fragrance of essential oils can be enjoyed without any extra equipment. Soak a cotton ball in essential oil and place either in a room or in a cupboard to scent the area. For maximum effect, place somewhere warm, such as behind a heater or fireplace. You can also sprinkle logs or twigs with lavender oil before placing them on the

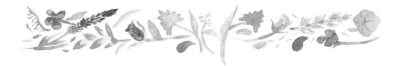

fire, or use rosemary on the wood in a barbecue for a wonderful permeating aroma. If you have a congested nose, a single drop of a suitable oil, such as cypress or eucalyptus, on a tissue or handkerchief can offer relief.

IMPORTANT

The extraction of essential oils is an extremely intensive process which can result in a rather expensive product, but a true oil is very concentrated and only requires a tiny amount to work its wonders. Be sure to buy your oils from a reliable informed supplier who can advise you if the oil has been blended. Although some essential oils, such as lavender, are safe for even the beginner to use, others are very strong and can be toxic if used undiluted.

Oils should be used under the guidance of a qualified herbalist or aromatherapist. This is particularly important if you suffer from high blood pressure, epilepsy, or a neural disorder, as some essential oils can aggravate these conditions. Similarly, certain oils should be avoided during pregnancy as they can trigger menstruation or miscarriage. If you have sensitive skin or suffer from allergies, consult an aromatherapist before using any essential oil. If in doubt, do a patch test first.

Frankincense

Boswellia thurifera • Boswellia carteri

DESCRIPTION AND HISTORY

Frankincense was one of the most highly prized substances of the ancient world. The three wise men who came to pay homage to the baby Jesus bore gifts of gold, frankincense and myrrh. At one time the Arabians from the south even had to pay an annual tribute in frankincense to the Persian king Darius. Revered as a holy perfume, this fragrant tree gum was most frequently burned as incense. The name "frankincense" in itself can be traced to 10th century France and means "luxuriant incense".

MEDICINAL

In ancient Egypt, frankincense was much prized as a skin tonic. Today, this beautifully scented essential oil is recognized for its decidedly restorative action, making it ideal for more mature skin. Aromatherapists use frankincense to treat respiratory complaints, for it has the effect of slowing and regulating the breathing. This calming property makes it a good nerve tonic — add a few drops to a warm bath if you want to relax — and also a useful aid for meditation.

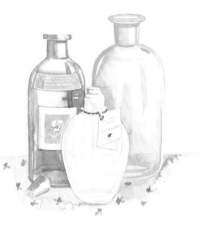

PROPERTIES

Nervine • respiratory • restorative • benefits the female system • rejuvenating • comforting

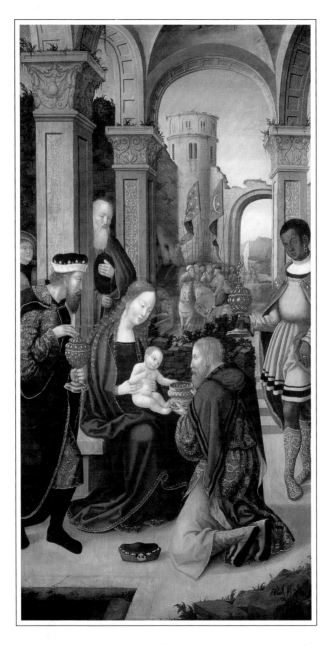

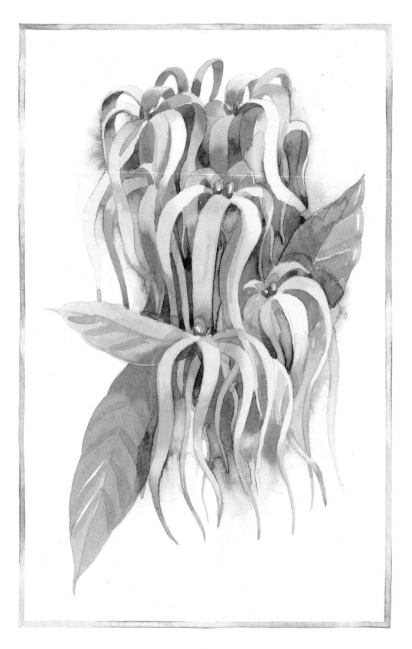

DESCRIPTION AND HISTORY

*T*he beautiful yellow flower of the tropical ylang ylang tree of Java, Indonesia, the Philippines, and Madagascar, is so exotic and its perfume is so extraordinary that it is known as the "flower of flowers". Essential oil of ylang ylang is extracted from the flowers by steam distillation.

MEDICINAL

The sweet heady scent of ylang ylang encompasses strong sensual and euphoric qualities, and the oil is heralded as an aphrodisiac. This essential oil is also renowned for its restorative powers and its relaxing effect on the nervous system. The oil is an antidepressant and may be used therapeutically to treat stress, frustration, anger, and shock. It can have a balancing effect on blood pressure and distressed breathing patterns. Although used in many cosmetics for its fragrance, ylang ylang is also included in preparations for its balancing and toning effect on skin.

PROPERTIES

Antiseptic • aphrodisiac • sedative • nervine

Ylang ylang

Cananga odorata

A BEAUTIFULLY SCENTED FACIAL CLEANSING OIL MAY BE MADE BY COMBINING ONE CUP OF APRICOT KERNEL OIL AND HALF A CUP OF WALNUT OIL WITH ONE TABLESPOON OF AVOCADO OIL AND EIGHT TO TEN DROPS OF YLANG YLANG OIL. POUR ALL THE OILS INTO A SCREW-TOP JAR AND SHAKE WELL. TO USE, POUR SOME OF THE OIL ONTO A PIECE OF COTTON WOOL AND GENTLY APPLY TO THE FACE USING UPWARD AND OUTWARD MOVEMENTS.

DESCRIPTION AND HISTORY

C loves are actually the unexpanded flower buds of the clove tree, produced almost as a monopoly in the country of Zanzibar. Best known as a spice, the same buds provide the aromatherapist with attar of cloves. Centuries before Christ, envoys to the Han court of China held clove oil in their mouths to freshen their breath during audiences with the emperor. In the 19th century, the oil was applied to gentlemen's handkerchiefs which were held to the nose to disguise the smell of filthy streets. It is still used in making soaps, perfumes, and cosmetics.

MEDICINAL

The ships that brought cloves to Europe from the East often carried a hidden cargo as well — exotic diseases. It is strange irony that the potent oil from the cloves was later to serve as a protective against the bubonic plague. Sponges impregnated with clove oil were held beneath the nostrils of patients, and doctors wore masks soaked in clove oil to protect them. Modern evidence suggests clove oil does indeed have important medical value as one of the most effective antiseptics known. It is good for treating infections, especially colds and flu, and is often an ingredient in commercially available mouthwashes and digestive tonics. Clove oil will also bring a welcome numbness if applied topically for a toothache or sore gums.

PROPERTIES

Antiseptic • antispasmodic • slightly aphrodisiac • analgesic • digestive • nervine • respiratory • carminative • warming

CAUTION

Avoid use during pregnancy.

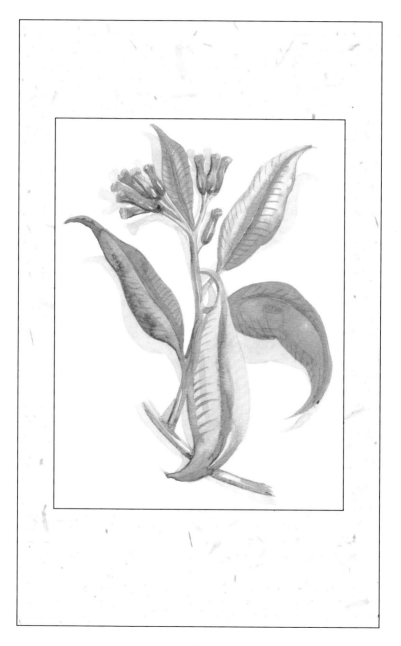

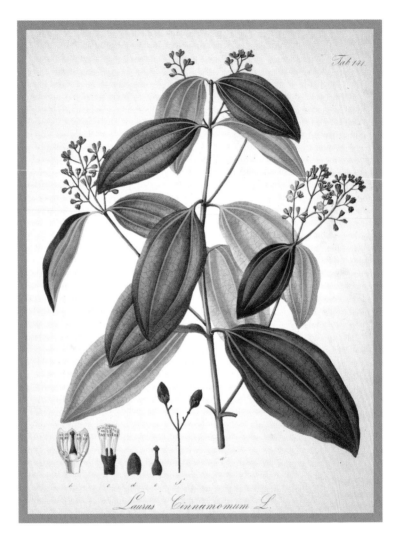

Laurus Cinnamomum L.

"If odours may worke satisfaction, they are so soveraigne in plants
and so comfortable that no confection of the apothecaries can equall
their excellent Vertue."

JOHN GERARD, THE HERBALL, 1597

The name cinnamon comes from the Malay *kayu manis*, meaning "sweet wood". With its soft and sweet aroma, cinnamon has been valued since ancient times. The Queen of Sheba gave cinnamon to King Solomon and it was one of the spices used to make holy ointment for the Tabernacle. The legendary phoenix was said to construct its magic pyre from cinnamon and myrrh.

It is not the fruit of this plant but the fragrant bark that is harvested for general use. The essential oil is distilled from the leaves and is used to perfume soaps, scents, and cosmetics. It is often included as an ingredient in toothpastes and is used to improve the taste of medicines.

Cinnamomum zeylanicum **Cinnamon**

MEDICINAL

Rich and spicy, cinnamon oil is very strongly aromatic and provides an effective remedy for flu, nausea, fatigue, and depression. The oil may be used to prepare a warming soothing rub for rheumatism.

PROPERTIES

Antiseptic • digestive • respiratory • tonifying for skin • aphrodisiac • haemostatic • astringent

CAUTION

Avoid use during pregnancy.

Neroli

Citrus aurantium

hy the oil of the orange blossom should be called neroli is a mystery. It is popularly thought that the oil was named after the 16th century Princess of Nerola in Italy, who used it extravagantly to scent her clothes and rooms. It is much used in perfumery, notably the production of Eau de Cologne. Neroli oil is extremely expensive, but the perfume is absolutely exquisite.

MEDICINAL

Neroli makes a wonderful facial oil and massage blend, helping to regenerate skin cells and improve skin elasticity. It is one of the most suitable essential oils to use for nervous tension, insomnia, and stress-related illnesses as it is has a very positive calming influence on mind and body. It is rumoured to have aphrodisiac properties, no doubt due to its deeply relaxing effect and its enticing scent.

PROPERTIES

Antibacterial • calming • healing for the skin • circulatory • nervine • digestive • sedative • antidepressant • aphrodisiac

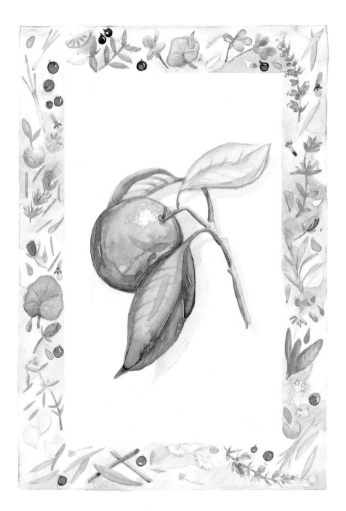

ORANGE

IN CONTRAST TO NEROLI, THE ESSENTIAL OIL OF ORANGE IS EXTRACTED FROM THE PEEL OF THE FRUIT. ITS AROMA TOO IS DELICIOUSLY SWEET WHICH PROMOTES A BRIGHT AND SOCIABLE MOOD. THE LIGHT, TANGY CRISPNESS OF THE OIL MAKES IT A DELIGHTFUL ROOM FRESHENER. ADD IT TO YOUR BATH FOR INSTANT REFRESHMENT. LIKE NEROLI, IT ALSO BENEFITS THE SKIN.

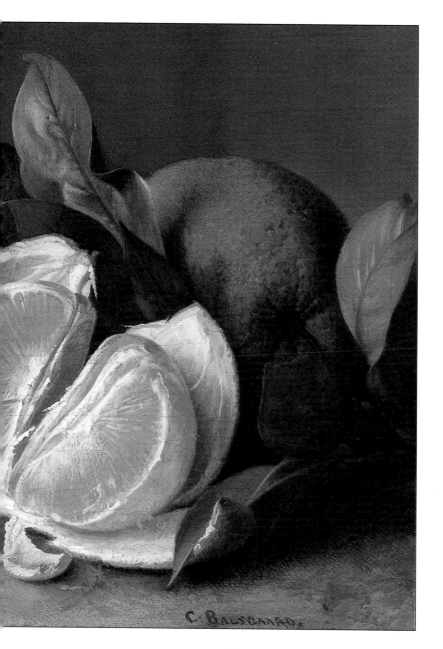

C. BALSCARAU.

DESCRIPTION AND HISTORY

Bergamot essential oil is derived from the fresh ripe peel of the bergamot orange after the juice has been extracted. It blends well with other oils to enhance their aroma and is most commonly used in commercial perfume manufacturing, being a key ingredient of Eau de Cologne.

MEDICINAL

Bergamot is a powerful antiseptic and may be diluted for treating skin or scalp conditions and for dressing wounds. It has a natural deodorizing effect, both as a breath freshener or as a personal deodorant. Depression and anxiety are effectively treated with this refreshing oil.

PROPERTIES

Respiratory • uplifting
• clarifying • antiseptic
• digestive • skin
and hair
treatment

A SWEET-SMELLING HERBAL PILLOW, DESIGNED TO RELAX EVEN THE MOST HARDENED INSOMNIAC, CAN BE MADE WITH EQUAL QUANTITIES OF DRIED ROSE BUDS AND ROSE GERANIUM LEAVES, SPRINKLED WITH BERGAMOT AND ROSE OIL.

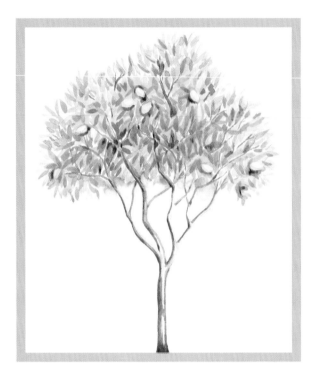

DESCRIPTION AND HISTORY

*T*he tangy lemon is one of the oldest and most useful natural cosmetics; it also has a long traditional use as a medicine. The plant was originally a native of south-eastern Asia until the Arabs brought the lemon to the Mediterranean in AD 1000. Some early Christian artists portrayed it as the fruit of the Tree of Knowledge which Eve ate before being expelled from Eden. Essential oil of lemon is derived from the rind of the fruit.

MEDICINAL

The Romans dosed pregnant women with lemon cordials, according to Pliny "... to stay flux and vomit". The fresh, sharply aromatic oil is still used to treat nausea and to stimulate the appetite. Use it also as a massage to aid circulation. The lemon's antiseptic properties are well-respected and make it effective in treating colds and sore throats and in controlling skin blemishes. The mild sedative action will reduce fever and ease indigestion. Most particularly, lemon oil helps to stimulate the body's own natural defences against infection.

Lemon oil may be used as a natural cosmetic. It has a wonderful toning effect, mild deodorant properties, and will provide a gentle exfoliant action. Use it as a rinse or in a bath to lighten hair or skin, as a tooth cleanser, or in a cooling lotion to soothe sunburn.

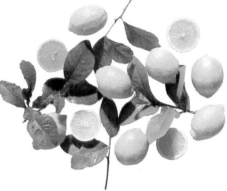

PROPERTIES

Antiseptic • physical stimulant • skin tonic • antibacterial • astringent • diuretic • circulatory • refreshing • cooling • uplifting

Citrus limonum **Lemon**

Myrrh

Commiphora myrrha

DESCRIPTION AND HISTORY

*T*he essential oil of myrrh is a highly aromatic oil which is distilled from the gum resin produced by the bark of the small Middle Eastern tree, *Commiphora myrrh*a. The oil has a deep golden colour and a sweet, camphor-like scent. Myrrh is mentioned often in the Bible and — with gold and frankincense — is perhaps best known as one of the gifts the three wise men brought to pay homage to the baby Jesus. Myrrh was one of the most highly prized substances of the ancient world and was much used in ancient religious ceremonies, primarily for embalming and devotional purposes. It was frequently burned as incense.

MEDICINAL

The early Greeks were aware of myrrh's power as an antiseptic and healing agent and they used it both externally to treat and disinfect wounds and skin problems, and internally for digestive upsets. Myrrh oil may be used as an antiseptic gargle and is very useful for dental problems, hence its use in many toothpastes.

PROPERTIES

Healing • digestive
• anti-inflammatory
• respiratory • tonic
• stimulating • antifungal
• astringent • antiseptic
• rejuvenating

CAUTION

Myrrh should be avoided by pregnant women.

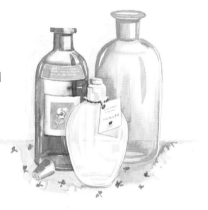

THE TEAR-SHAPED DROPS OF THE GUM
RESIN FROM COMMIPHORA MYRRHA ARE
THOUGHT TO EXPLAIN THE ORIGIN OF THE
TREE'S NAME IN MYTH. WHEN MYRRHA,
A YOUNG GREEK GIRL, REFUSED TO
WORSHIP AHPRODITE, THE GODDESS
OF LOVE WAS SO MUCH
AGGRIEVED THAT SHE
THREATENED TO KILL THE
GIRL. THE OTHER GODS
TOOK PITY ON MYRRHA
AND CHANGED HER
INTO THIS TREE
WHICH HAS "WEPT"
EVERMORE.

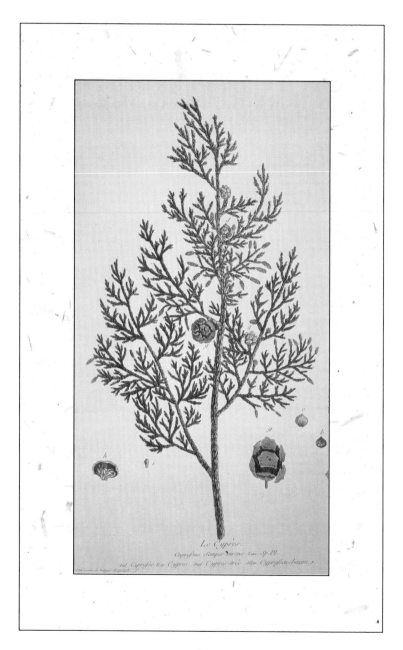

Le Cyprès.

Cupressus Semper virens Linn. Sp. Pl.

ital. Cipresso ; esp. Cyprès ; angl. Cyprus-tree ; allem. Cypressen-baum .

Cypress

Cupressus sempervirens

*a*ccording to Greek myth, the mournful-looking cypress tree was formed from the body of a hunter named Cyparissus, who killed one of Apollo's stags by mistake and was overcome by guilt and regret for his action. The cypress tree also came to represent the gods of the underworld in Greek mythology. Branches from the trees were placed in the graves of the newly dead, for they were thought to ease a person's passage into the afterlife. Tibetans used cypress as a purification incense. The resinous, woody oil is distilled from the leaves, cones, and flowers of the tree.

MEDICINAL

Cypress oil contains several strongly aromatic principles which work together as an effective tonic for nervous disorders, by acting as a sedative on the nervous and respiratory systems. The oil is a common ingredient in many commercial preparations used for the treatment of colds, bronchitis, or flu. Try a few drops on a pillow or handkerchief to relieve nasal congestion. Cypress oil is also a powerful astringent and a natural therapist may prescribe it for either external use in healing wounds and balancing problem skin, or internally for circulatory problems. Added to a bath, cypress oil can relieve heavy aching legs and swollen ankles. Alternatively, massage the legs with a blend made from a carrier oil to which two or three drops of cypress oil have been added. The oil is also a good natural deodorant.

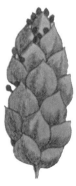

PROPERTIES

Balances the female system • stimulating • circulatory • respiratory • decongestive • head-clearing • antispasmodic • gently diuretic • refreshing

CAUTION

Avoid use of cypress oil if you suffer from high blood pressure.

DESCRIPTION AND HISTORY

T he eucalypt was dubbed the "fever tree" because the strong balsamic odours were supposed to increase the healthfulness of the swampy areas where the trees seemed to thrive. Baron Ferdinand von Mueller of the Botanical Gardens in Melbourne, Australia, was the first to suggest that eucalyptus oil had medicinal qualities. He sent seeds to Algiers where it was found that not only did the trees exude a refreshing and antiseptic aroma in marshy, illness-riddled districts, but the trees' roots helped dry out the water-logged soil. In Sicily, eucalyptus trees were similarly planted as a malaria preventive. The medicinal qualities of eucalyptus oil were given the official seal of approval in 1885 in the British Pharmacopeia.

MEDICINAL

Eucalypts are among the most aromatic plants in the world and the sharply scented oil given off by the leaves has powerful healing, disinfectant, and antiseptic uses. Well known for its use in inhalants to treat respiratory conditions, the oil is also useful for wounds and insect bites. Cooling to the body, a compress made from a cool dilution of eucalyptus oil can relieve fever and skin irritations. Used in vapourizers or room sprays the oil helps cleanse and disinfect the air.

PROPERTIES

Head-clearing • refreshing • stimulating • uplifting • invigorating • respiratory • decongestive • antiseptic • cooling • cleansing • anti-inflammatory • antispasmodic • analgesic

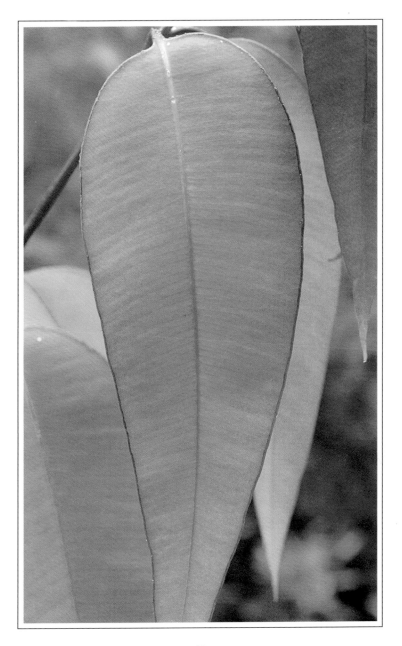

TAKE LENGTHS OF THICK PARCHMENT-STYLE PAPER (WALLPAPER IS IDEAL) AND CUT TO FIT THE INSIDES OF DRAWERS. COVER WITH DRIED JASMINE FLOWERS, ROLL UP AND SEAL IN PLASTIC BAGS. AFTER SIX WEEKS, THE PAPER WILL HAVE ABSORBED THE PERFUME. TO INTENSIFY THE FRAGRANCE, DAB A FEW DROPS OF JASMINE OIL ONTO A COTTON BALL AND WIPE AROUND THE INSIDE OF EACH DRAWER BEFORE SETTING THE PAPER INSIDE.

DESCRIPTION AND HISTORY

*g*n India, jasmine is revered as sacred to Vishnu and the flowers are often strung into garlands for votive offerings in religious ceremonies. Those same flowers exude an exotic and heady fragrance that stirs the senses. Cleopatra used oil of jasmine to woo Mark Antony. It is little wonder that to the aromatherapist the petals of the jasmine are as precious as those of the rose. The essential oil is extracted through the time-consuming process of enfleurage. A costly oil, jasmine is an ingredient of many fine perfumes.

MEDICINAL

Jasmine essential oil is highly esteemed for treating problems of the nervous system, dispersing depression, tension, listlessness, and fear. The oil is often included in natural skin care products for its smoothing and softening effect on skin, and it is useful in preventing scarring by increasing the skin's elasticity.

PROPERTIES

Relaxing • uplifting • positive effect on the female system • aphrodisiac • strong sensual stimulant

Jasmine

Jasminum grandiflorum • Jasminum officinale

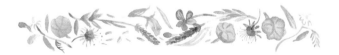

".. the city was like snow at night, and was fragrant everywhere. The flowers were used in making perfumes and scented oils to rub on the body. Indeed, everyone had the delicious scent about them ..."

CHI HAN, RECORDS OF THE PLANTS OF SOUTHERN CHINA, 3RD CENTURY AD

DESCRIPTION AND HISTORY

O ne of the oldest known essential oils, cedarwood was an important ingredient in the medicine, cosmetics, and perfumery of the ancient Egyptians. The attar of cedar grew in popularity in the 19th century when it was used as an ingredient in "cold cream soap" and, diluted with spirits of wine, was used to saturate handkerchiefs.

MEDICINAL

The strong balsam-like fragrance of cedarwood essential oil makes it useful as an all-round tonic and stimulant. It can thus be used to treat problems concerned with a sluggish system, particularly respiratory and skin complaints. Cedarwood is thought to possess aphrodisiac properties, presumably because of its exhilarating scent.

PROPERTIES

Antiseptic • digestive • astringent • tonifying • calming • aphrodisiac • harmonizing • strengthening

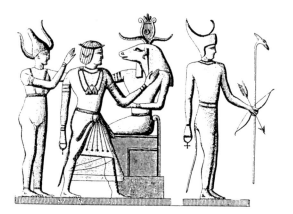

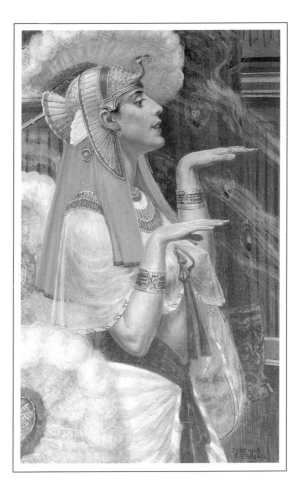

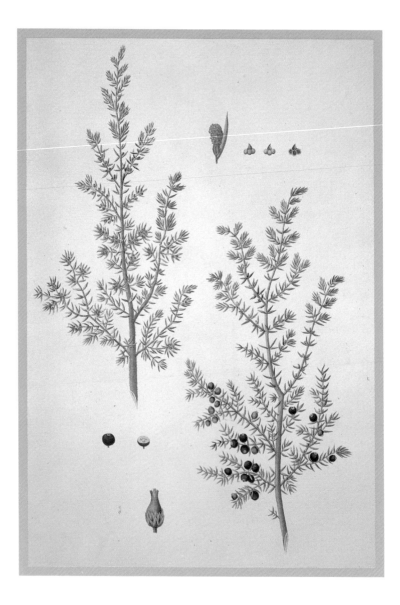

Juniperus communis **Juniper**

*J*uniper has long been regarded as a magical herb. In the Middle Ages, a juniper bush would be planted by the door in the belief that this kept witches away. During times of plague the branches were burnt to ward off disease. As recently as World War II, French nurses burned juniper in field army hospitals to disinfect the air. The ancient Egyptians used juniper oil in the embalming process but these days the plant is best known as the source of gin. The essential oil of juniper should not be confused with juniper oil; the latter may be cheaper, but is usually made by distilling the leaves and twigs, while the essential, and most effective, oil is made from the berries only.

MEDICINAL

Known since ancient times for its antiseptic and diuretic qualities, juniper was described by 17th century English herbalist Nicolas Culpeper as "provoking urine exceedingly".
In addition, Culpeper prescribed juniper for "cough, shortness of breath" and "to give safe and speedy delivery to women with child". Juniper has a marked effect on the digestive system, the female system, and the circulatory system — whether used in a massage blend or prescribed orally. By association, problem skin can benefit from the oil. It serves as a useful general tonic — a few drops of the oil in a warm bath or in a massage oil is helpful in treating sleeplessness and stress.

PROPERTIES

Nervine • diuretic • analgesic • muscle relaxant
• cleansing • toning • balancing • digestive
• stimulates appetite • circulatory • carminative

Bay

Laurus nobilis

DESCRIPTION AND HISTORY

According to Classical legend, the bay tree was sacred to Apollo, the god of medicine. Apollo was said to have been infatuated with the pretty nymph Daphne, but she did not return his affection. She begged the gods to help her escape, and they changed her into a bay tree. Heartbroken Apollo took the tree as his emblem, hence the custom of bestowing bay wreaths on heroes, artists, and emperors.

From very early times, bay was considered a potent magical herb. The Delphic oracle was said to hold bay leaves between her teeth when prophesising events. Medieval "wise women" made talismans from bay to avert "the evil eye". In 1652, herbalist Nicolas Culpeper averred that " ... neither witch nor devil, thunder nor lightning will hurt a man where a bay tree is". The leaves and berries of bay yield the oil, by distillation.

MEDICINAL

Bay leaves, berries, and bark have all been attributed with medicinal qualities. The pungent smell was thought to repel infection, so physicians would rub their hands with the oil after ministering to a sick patient. During outbreaks of plague, residents of ancient Rome were advised to burn bay oil in public places. The aromatic oil has long been used as a soothing rub for arthritis and rheumatism, with 17th century herbalist Nicolas Culpeper recommending it "for all griefes of the jointes". An aromatherapist may prescribe it to relieve earache or to lower blood pressure.

PROPERTIES

• Soothing • antibacterial • circulatory • relaxing • anti-inflammatory.

CAUTION

Avoid external use of bay if you have extremely sensitive skin as it may provoke a rash.

"Bay serveth to adorn the House of God, as well as of Man; to procure warmth, comfort and strength, to the limmes of men and of women by bathings and anoyntings."

JOHN PARKINSON

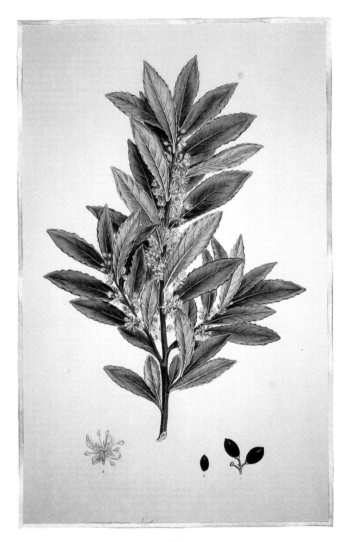

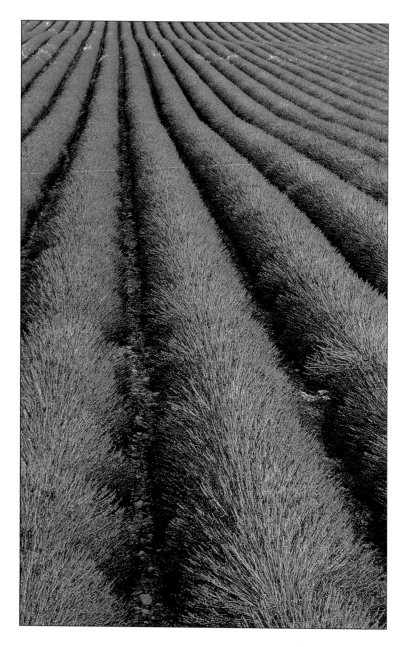

*D*uring Elizabethan times the aromatic oil of lavender was rubbed into oak furniture to give a high gloss. Apart from the enjoyable scent, lavender provided a powerful weapon against moths, fleas, silverfish, and flies. Commercial perfume houses still use essential oil of lavender as the basic ingredient of many fragrances.

MEDICINAL

Essential oil of lavender is the most widely used and versatile healing oil. Not only is it extremely effective, it is also very easy to use and is the only oil that can be safely applied undiluted to the skin. Dr Gattefosse — one of the founders of the science of aromatherapy — was the first to pinpoint lavender's ability to restore skin health. The oil may be used with great success to treat skin disorders, preventing scarring and promoting rapid healing. Lavender oil is also one of the stronger antiseptic oils and is included in a variety of cosmetic aids such as mouthwash, skin tonic, and eye-lotion, in addition to making a natural insect repellent. The oil provides a soothing rub for patients suffering from arthritis and rheumatism, a good inhalant for respiratory problems and fainting, and a relieving compress for headaches. The balancing properties of lavender can correct emotional problems and feelings of instability. Its calming effect will induce a restful sleep — try a drop of lavender oil on your pillow or into an evening bath.

PROPERTIES

Head-clearing • respiratory • skin healing • nervine • muscle relaxant • digestive • sedative • calming • balancing • analgesic • antiseptic • antibacterial • decongestive • antidepressant

Lavandula officinalis *Lavender*

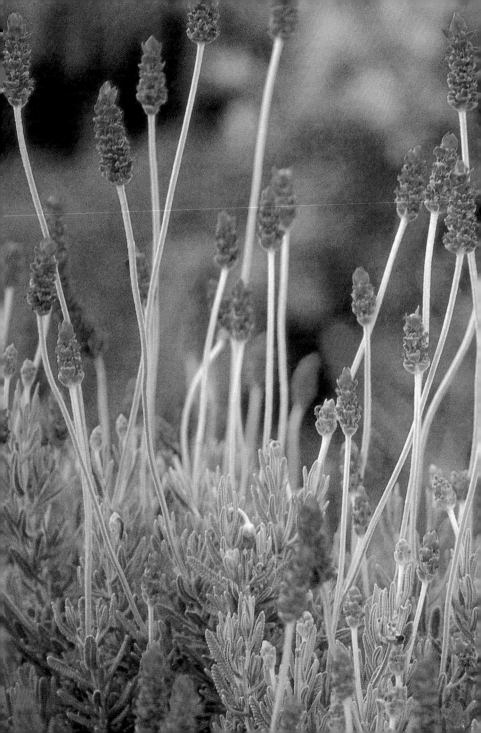

"I judge that the flowres of lavender quilted in a cap and dayly worne are good for all diseases of the head that come of a cold cause and that they comfort the braine very well."

WILLIAM TURNER, A NEW HERBALL (1551)

Chamomile

Matricaria chamomilla (German) • *Anthemis nobilis (Roman)*

DESCRIPTION AND HISTORY

*T*here are many different types of chamomile, all distinguished by their pretty daisy-like flowers and bright green feathery leaves which give off a strong fruity scent when crushed. The oils of German and Roman chamomile, distilled from the plants' flowering tops, share similar soothing properties.

Chamomile has long been cultivated as a medicinal herb and, no doubt due to its healing prowess, it was even considered sacred. In 1656, John Parkinson wrote: "Camomill is put to divers and sundry uses, both for pleasure and profit, both for the sick and the sound, in bathing to comfort and strengthen the sound and to ease pains in the diseased". Even before this, the Egyptian priests dedicated the plant to Ra, their sun god and India's Ayurvedic physicians also used it for digestive upsets, cramps, and fever.

MEDICINAL

Chamomile oil became so popular in Germany as a medicine that it was known as *alles zutruat* meaning "capable of anything". The soothing oil has been variously prescribed to speed healing, calm inflammation and allergies, and treat burns and bruises, earache, neuralgia, abcesses, and toothache.

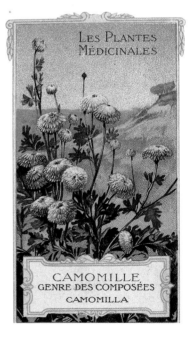

LES PLANTES MÉDICINALES

CAMOMILLE
GENRE DES COMPOSÉES
CAMOMILLA

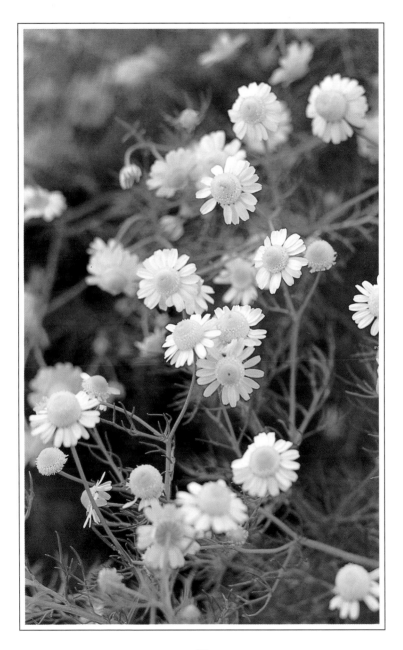

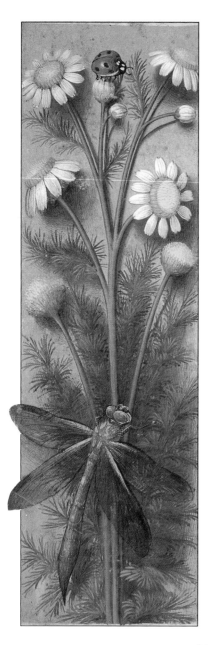

Chamomile's fragrance has a definite calming effect — a steam inhalation can assuage insomnia and hysteria. It is also a useful herb for natural beauty care. The early Vikings are said to have rinsed their hair with an infusion of chamomile, thus enhancing their blondness. Chamomile oil may be used as a hair conditioner. It is a very effective treatment for skin disorders — try adding a few drops of the oil to bath water to ease dry or sunburned skin.

PROPERTIES

Soothing • mildly antiseptic • analgesic • calming • muscle relaxant • digestive • balancing for the female system

CAUTION

Should not be used in the early months of pregnancy.

"To comfort the braine,
smel to camomill ... wash
measurably, sleep reasonably;
delight to hear melody
and singing ..."

RAM'S LITTLE DODOEN, 1606

TO MAKE OYLE OF CAMOMILE — TAKE OYLE A PINT AND
A HALFE, AND THREE OUNCES OF CAMOMILE FLOWERS
DRYED ONE DAY AFTER THEY BE GATHERED. THEN PUT
THE OYLE AND THE FLOWERS IN A GLASSE AND STOP THE
MOUTH CLOSE AND SET IT INTO THE SUN BY THE SPACE
OF FORTY DAYS.

The Good Housewife's Handbook, 1588

Tea Tree Hair Tonic

MIX THE FOLLOWING INGREDIENTS
TOGETHER AND WARM FOR A
STIMULATING MASSAGE TREATMENT
FOR SCALP AND HAIR PROBLEMS.

5 drops tea tree oil
5 drops eucalyptus oil
$^1/_3$ cup (100 ml) pure alcohol
$^1/_3$ cup (100 ml) castor oil

DESCRIPTION AND HISTORY

*T*he early European colonists of Australia and New Zealand used the pungent leaves of this plant to make tea, hence the common name. Not only was this a most pleasant drink, it was used by the explorer Captain Cook to overcome scurvy among his men. The Australian Aborigines already used poultices of pulped tea tree leaves to heal wounds. Oil is obtained from the leaves via steam distillation

MEDICINAL

The fresh lemony scent of tea tree oil is very pleasant, having a marvellous cleansing and head-clearing effect. It is renowned as an antifungal and antiseptic treatment, and may be used directly to treat skin conditions and wounds or as an inhalant to treat respiratory infections. Diluted and applied topically, it is very effective in correcting bacterial imbalances in the female system. Tea tree oil also serves as an efficient natural insect repellant and is often included in cleansing preparations and insect collars for cats and dogs; use the oil domestically in a burner to repel mosquitoes.

PROPERTIES

Antiseptic • antifungal • digestive • skin healing • antibacterial • respiratory • decongestive

Melaleuca alternifolia **Tea tree**

49

Peppermint

Mentha piperita

DESCRIPTION AND HISTORY

ℳ ints are recorded in the Ebers papyrus, the world's oldest surviving medical text, and are frequently mentioned in the Bible. The Greeks and Romans crowned themselves with mint for banquets and put bunches on the table in the hope of warding off drunkenness. Ending a meal with a sprig of mint to help the digestion and sweeten the breath is a very ancient custom, culminating in the widespread popularity of "after dinner mints" today. Mint was used for scenting bath water, being thought to "strengthen the sinews" at the same time. Peppermint is the most widely used mint. The oil is distilled from the leaves and flowering tips of the plants.

MEDICINAL

Greek and Roman herbalists prescribed mint for just about everything, from hiccups to leprosy. English herbalist Nicolas Culpeper wrote: "Mint is very profitable to the stomach". Peppermint oil, particularly as an inhalation, relieves nausea and respiratory problems, and aids digestion. A gargle made with the oil will assist these conditions and freshen the breath. A mild washing water, made by adding a few drops of peppermint oil to distilled water, is a cooling lotion for those with sensitive skin. The cooling effect extends to the emotions, clearing the mind. Rats and mice detest the invigorating aroma making rags soaked in peppermint oil a very effective deterrent of vermin.

PROPERTIES

Digestive • carminative • respiratory • anti-inflammatory • balancing to the female system • cooling (and warming) • clearing • muscle relaxant

Peppermint Travel Pillow

TO EASE APPREHENSION AND MOTION
SICKNESS MAKE A SOFT NECK CUSHION
AND FILL IT WITH:

$1/4$ cup (50 g) peppermint

1 tablespoon (15 g) mint-scented pelargonium

$1/4$ cup (50 g) lemon verbena

$1/4$ cup (50 g) lavender

1 tablespoon crushed lemon zest

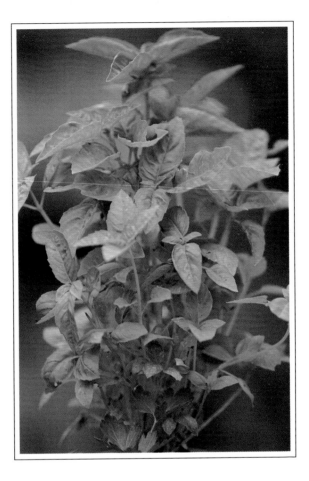

The smell of basil is good for the heart and the head, that the seed cureth
the infirmities of the heart, taketh away sorrowfulnesse which cometh of
melancholy ... maketh a man merrie and glad."

JOHN GERARD, 1597

S un-loving basil has been cultivated for at least 4000 years and, through the ages, has had a somewhat contradictory reputation. It was native to India — where it was a sacred herb, believed to protect against evil — and spread from there to ancient Greece, where it became a symbol of hostility and insanity. Today's French phrase *semer le basilic*, meaning "to curse", is derived from this. Basil appears to have reached Europe by the mid 16th century where it was used both as a strewing herb and as a medicine, and where the oil was used to scent snuff. There are now around 150 varieties of basil in the world, the oil being obtained from the flowering tops and leaves.

Ocimum basilicum **Basil**

MEDICINAL

Seventeenth century herbalist Jacques Tournefourt was convinced that smelling basil would cause venomous scorpions to breed in a person's brain, and this tale — understandably — meant that basil was viewed askance by physicians for some time. Despite this, basil and its oil has been used widely as a medicinal herb, primarily for settling an upset stomach. John Gerard recommended basil "to procure a merrie and cheerful heart", which was probably a reference to its tonic effects. The oil has a clarifying effect on the mind and aids concentration. It is also useful for soothing skin abrasions.

PROPERTIES

Digestive • respiratory • soothing • calming • muscle relaxant • head-clearing • uplifting • clarifying • aphrodisiac • mentally stimulating

CAUTION

Avoid use during pregnancy.

Marjoram

Origanum majorana

DESCRIPTION AND HISTORY

Traditionally used to make wreaths with which to crown newlywed couples for luck, marjoram was also used medicinally for a number of complaints — from digestive disorders to curing toothache. It was a valuable strewing herb. John Gerard wrote marjoram was "excellent good against all cold diseases of the brain and head". Early Greek physicians found it an antidote to poisoning, snake venom, and hemlock. The Romans used it widely for settling the stomach and for dizziness. Nicolas Culpeper recommended marjoram as "... an excellent remedy for the braine and other parts of the body", adding that a dressing of marjoram and honey would help reduce "the marks of blows". Marjoram oil is extracted from the leaves and flowering tops of the plant by means of steam distillation.

MEDICINAL

This strongly aromatic oil may be added to a carrier oil and used as a gentle rub for muscular aches, bruises, sprains, and arthritic pain. It also has a very strong effect on the female system. The oil is the most strongly sedative of all essential oils and can quieten excessively heightened emotions and offer sleep to the insomniac, especially if enjoyed in a warming bath.

PROPERTIES

- antispasmodic • carminative
- respiratory • nervine
- calming • muscle relaxant
- digestive • sedative

CAUTION

Pregnant women should not use marjoram oil.

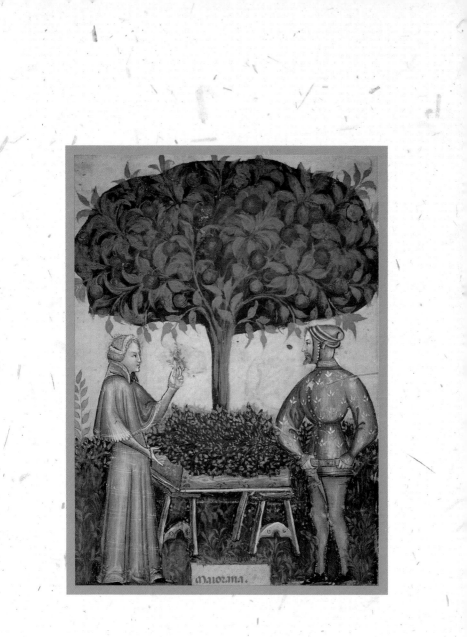

MAIORANA.

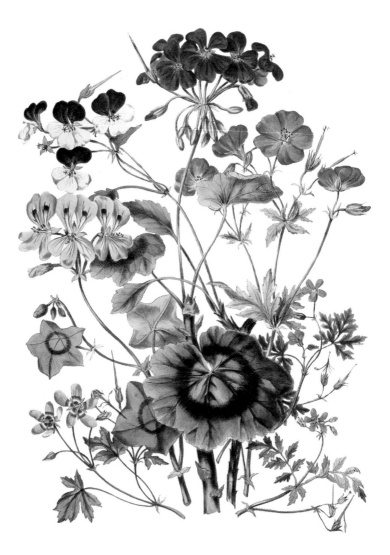

DESCRIPTION AND HISTORY

*T*hese scented flowering plants were discovered in the Cape Province of South Africa and brought to England in the time of Charles I. As potted plants in Victorian homes they would often be placed up the side of stairs so the women's long skirts would brush against them in passing, thus releasing the perfume. The essential oil of geranium is mostly obtained from the leaves, via steam distillation, and has developed into one of the most widely used essential oils in perfumery and cosmetic production.

MEDICINAL

Essential oil of geranium is acclaimed by aromatherapists as a good "all rounder". It may be prescribed for emotional disorders, to treat skin conditions, and as an insect repellent. Geranium oil is astringent and refreshing, and its rich sweet aroma makes it a popular choice in massage treatments and footbaths. Its principal effect is on the blood, making it a wonderful relief to tired and aching limbs. Use it in a vapourizer to treat respiratory complaints, or as a gargle to treat a sore throat. A balancing oil, it is invaluable for skin care, for the female system (especially for new mothers), and for harmonizing the emotions.

PROPERTIES

Antiseptic • antidepressant • anti-inflammatory • diuretic • balancing • tonifying • warming • refreshing • relaxing • harmonizing

Pelargonium graveolens **Geranium**

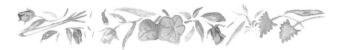

Anise
Pimpinella anisum

DESCRIPTION AND HISTORY

*a*lthough a native of Egypt, anise was grown in the old herb gardens of Europe as early as the 14th century. Best known as a culinary herb, it has an aromatic, penetrating sweetness which makes it an important ingredient in the manufacture of alcoholic beverages, such as Pernod. It also provides the distinctive taste in cough lozenges, some cordials, and tea blends. Manufacturers of perfumes, cosmetics, even toothpastes and insect repellents make use of this essential oil. The oil is extracted from the seeds via distillation.

MEDICINAL

Anise is one of the best-known digestive herbs; even in Roman times the seeds were chewed after rich meals. It is not surprising that the oil and the seeds are still both used in preparations to sweeten the breath and alleviate indigestion. The oil is also credited with being quite a strong antiseptic and possessing other medicinal properties that help to soothe coughs and headaches.

PROPERTIES

Digestive • head-clearing • warming • clarifying • respiratory • muscle relaxant

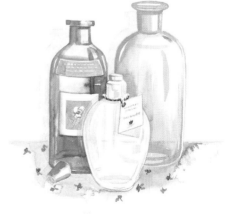

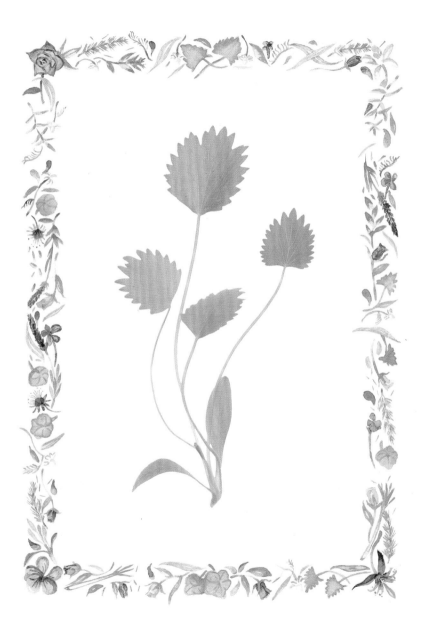

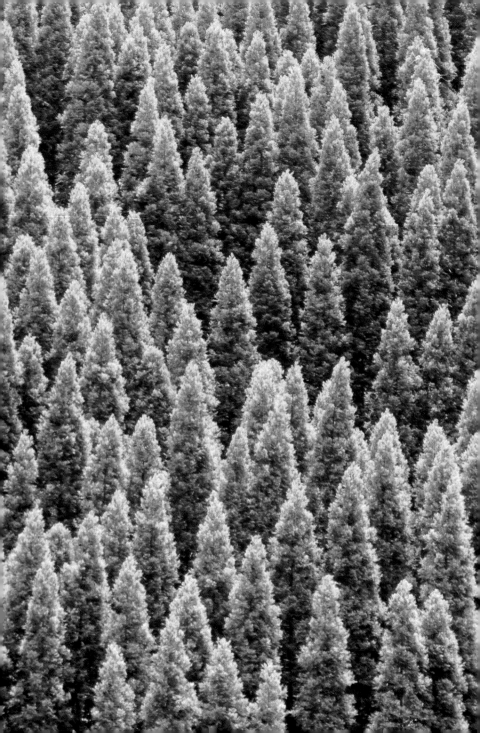

DESCRIPTION AND HISTORY

*T*he clean, fresh smell of pine oil is a familiar, everday aroma as it is used extensively in soaps and bath preparations, as well as household cleaning products, both for its scent and its antiseptic propetries. Essential oil of pine is distilled from the resins and needles of pine trees, of which there are over 100 varieties.

MEDICINAL

Essential oil of pine may be used internally or externally. Pine oil is a powerful antiseptic, probably best known for its effectiveness in treating infections of the respiratory system. The ancient Arab physician, Avicenna, prescribed it as an inhalation and poultice for a patient suffering from pneumonia. The oil has a stimulating effect on the circulation, making it warming rub for muscular pain. This invigorating quality will help treat lethargy and listlessness.

PROPERTIES

Respiratory • antiseptic • nervine • deodorant • stimulating

CAUTION

Pine oil should not be used in the bath by persons with sensitive skin, as it can cause skin irritation.

Pinus sylvestris **Pine**

Patchouli

Pogostemon patchouli

DESCRIPTION AND HISTORY

This essential oil is distilled from the dried branches of the bushy patchouli, a member of the lavender family, originating in Bengal, India. Patchouli came to Europe by an odd route. In Victorian England, there was a craze for wearing cashmere shawls from India and when they were packed for transportation to England, a whiff of patchouli always clung to them, starting the fashion for the scent. Patchouli was also used to give Indian ink its characteristic scent and dried patchouli leaves were laid amongst linen for their moth-repellent properties. The oil has a strong and persistent smell and is often used as a fixative in commercial perfume production or to mask over-strong aromas in cosmetics.

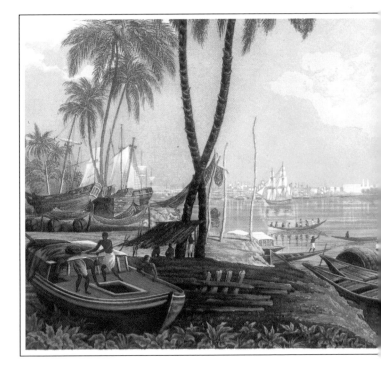

MEDICINAL

Patchouli oil is useful as an antiseptic, particularly as a first aid treatment for minor burns as it has an anti-inflammatory effect. Add several drops to a warm bath along with several spoonfuls of almond oil to soothe dry or irritated skin. The oil also works on irritated nerves, calming anxiety with its strongly earthy scent. This sensual, musky aroma is attributed with powers as an aphrodisiac.

PROPERTIES

Nervine • anti-inflammatory
• aphrodisiac • sedative • relaxing

"If the day and night are such that you greet them with joy and life emits a fragrance like flowers and sweet scented herbs — that is your success. All nature is your congratulations."

HENRY DAVID THOREAU

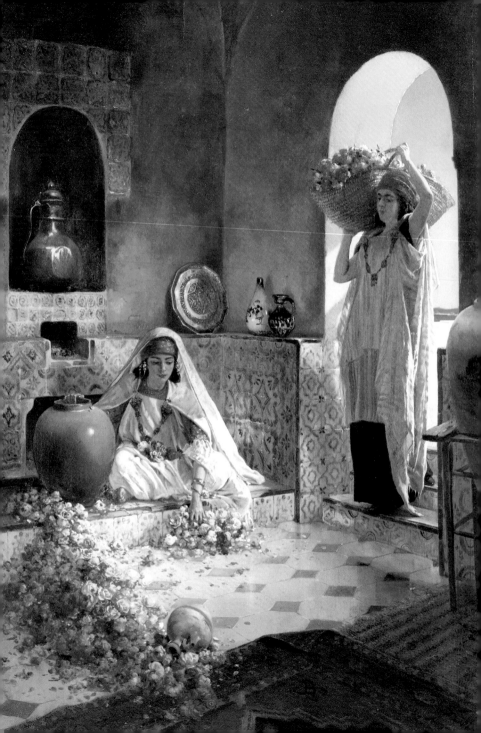

DESCRIPTION AND HISTORY

he "queen of essential oils" is one of the most prized and most valuable — it takes the petals of 30 damask roses to make one drop of Rose otto essential oil. The rose is the mystical symbol of love and romance, and its oil is thought to be an aphrodisiac. Legend has it that the Mogul prince, Jehangir, ordered roses to be floated in every canal running through the royal gardens to celebrate his wedding. His new wife, running her hands through the scented water, was fascinated to notice that a fragrant oil clung to her fingers and her doting husband ordered it bottled as a tribute to her.

MEDICINAL

Rose oil is probably best loved for its marvellously feminine and sensual fragrance. Therapeutically, this scent does have a potent anti-depressant effect and may be used, via face and body massage, skin care, baths, or vapourizers to treat nervousness, sadness, or long-term stress. Rose oil is often included in cosmetic creams for its refreshing and mild tonic effect on sensitive skin. Diluted in distilled water, rose oil may be used to soak compresses for tired or inflamed eyes. The oil is also an excellent remedy for disorders of the female system.

PROPERTIES

Antibacterial • balancing • astringent • antiseptic • antidepressant • anti-inflammatory • aphrodisiac • digestive

Rosa damascena (Rose otto) • Rosa centifolia (Rose absolute) **Rose**

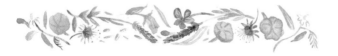

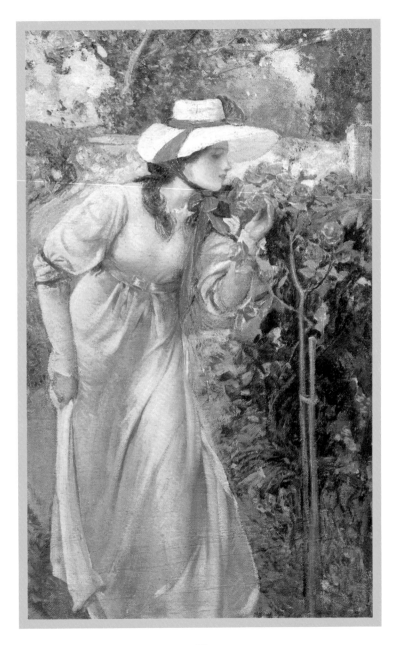

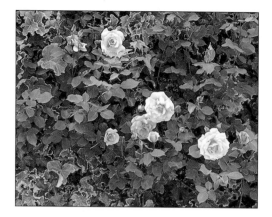

"To Make Oyle of Roses — Take of oyle
eighteen ounces, the buds of Roses (the
white ends of them cut away) three
ounces, lay the Roses abroad in the
shadow four and twenty houres, then put
them in a glass to the oyle, and stop the
glasse close, and set it in the sunne for
at least forty days."

John Partridge,
The Treasurie of Hidden Secrets and
Commodious Conceits, 1586

Rosemary

Rosmarinus officinalis

Rosemary has long been regarded as a preserver of youth — just smelling the plant was thought "to keep thee youngly". In Classical times, it became known as the herb of fidelity, love, and abiding friendship, and was bound into wedding wreaths and planted on graves. Bunches of rosemary were burned during times of plague in a bid to ward off infection, and judges and jury members held sprigs of rosemary when attending the courtroom to dispel any "jail fever" the criminal may have brought with him. The French hung rosemary in hospitals as a kind of healing incense and, as recently as World War II, the leaves were burned in field army hospitals for their antiseptic and purifying effect. Essential oil of rosemary is distilled from the flowering tops and leaves of the plants.

MEDICINAL

Rosemary was first noted as having preservative qualities centuries ago, when meat was wrapped in crushed rosemary leaves to stop it from spoiling. Rosemary oil has since been used in many preparations to ease the processes of ageing. Herbalists recommend it for hair care and suggest scalp massage with the oil to prevent premature baldness. Treat bad breath with a gargle made by adding a few drops of the oil to distilled water. With its powerful aroma, rosemary oil is an effective inhalant and decongestant, and a strengthening massage rub for muscles. This is the most stimulating of oils, enhancing memory, concentration, and clear thinking.

PROPERTIES

Invigorating • digestive • nervine • respiratory • circulatory • muscular • uplifting • stimulating

"... boyle the leves in white wine and wasshe thy face therewith ... thou shall have a fayre face ... wash thyself and thou shalt waxe shiny."

THE LEECH BOOK OF BALD

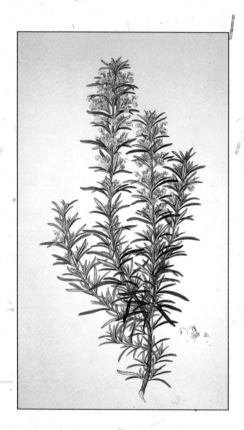

"For the sickly, take this wort rosemary, pound it with oil, smear the sickly one, wonderfully thou healest him."

SAXON HERBAL

"How can a man die who has sage in his garden?"

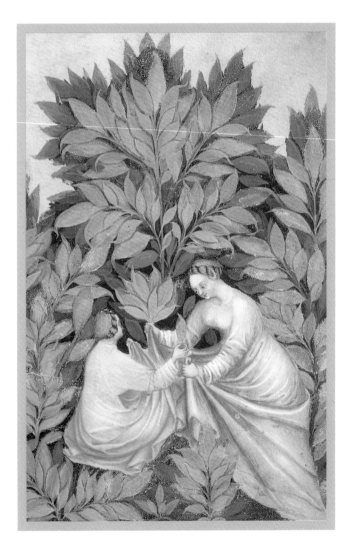

his very ancient herb has been held in high repute as a culinary and medicinal plant since Classical times. Its botanical name derives from the Latin "I save". The Greek physician Dioscorides wrote of it as "Sage the Saviour" and recommended it to ease headaches and nervous tension, and for a number of internal complaints. Sage oil is still extracted from the plant's leaves using traditional methods which have changed little over the centuries. The leaves are spread out to dry naturally in the hot sun on racks before they are distilled. Accordingly, sage oil is often slightly more expensive than most other essential oils.

Sage

Salvia officinalis

MEDICINAL

Sage has been used to treat all manner of malady. Essential oil of sage has an astringent and cooling effect, so it may be used as a spring tonic, a blood cleanser, and to promote the appetite, cool a fever, ease headaches, and heal skin conditions or wounds. Use diluted in distilled water as a gargle and mouthwash. It is an extremely effective natural deodorant and antiperspirant and can be burnt in a sick room to help cleanse and purify the air. Once widely used as as a remedy for "the ague" or rheumatism, massaging with the oil helps ease nervous and muscular tension or pain.

PROPERTIES

Diuretic • analgesic • antiseptic • nervine • relaxing

CAUTION

Avoid use during pregnancy.

DESCRIPTION AND HISTORY

The importance of Clary sage as a medicinal herb is evident in the origins of its name — "clary" is condensed from "clear-eye", the Old English name for this plant that was used safely and effectively to heal eye problems. In Germany it is known as Muscatel sage because of its use in the production of some wines and vermouths — it is thought to have intoxicating properties. Along with bergamot oil, clary sage oil is a key ingredient of Eau de Cologne and lavender toilet water. It is obtained from the flowering tops of the plants via steam distillation. Although related, this is a completely different oil from common sage (*Salvia officinalis*).

MEDICINAL

Clary sage has an astringent and tonic action, helping to stimulate the digestion, calm fevers, and produce a wonderfully cooling effect on the skin. For this reason, it may be included in cosmetic preparations to cleanse the skin, particularly if dry or sensitive. The oil has a marked relaxing effect and may be used to treat stress, high blood pressure, depression, and anxiety. It is also excellent for the female system.

PROPERTIES

Soothing • anti-inflammatory • calming • astringent • tonifying • warming • relaxing • uplifting

MAKE A SOOTHING EYE COMPRESS BY SOAKING PIECES OF CLEAN LINT OR COTTON IN COOLED BOILED WATER TO WHICH SEVERAL DROPS OF CLARY SAGE ESSENTIAL OIL HAVE BEEN ADDED. LAY THE COMPRESS OVER YOUR EYES FOR TEN MINUTES WHILE LYING DOWN AND RELAXING.

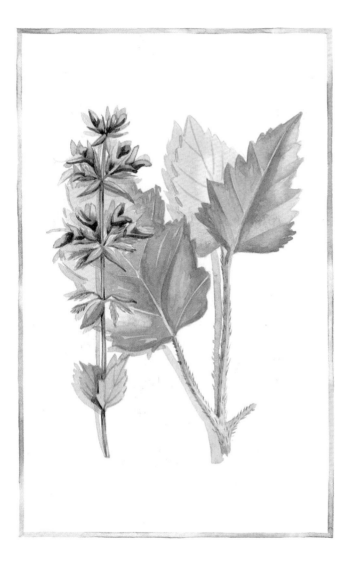

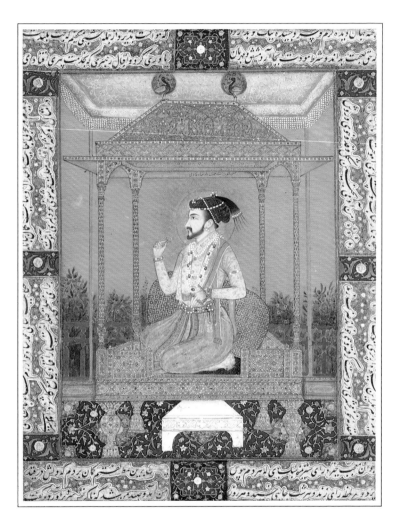

*T*his exotic essential oil captures the mystique of Asia where it forms part of Ayurveda, the Indian system of healing. Sandalwood oil was used in the embalming and funeral rites for Singhalese princes, and still plays an important part in Hindu marriages. It is burned on a sacred fire within the marriage tent so that its fumes surround the bridal couple. The oil is also burned as incense. In Burma, it is a custom on the last day of the year for women to sprinkle passersby with a mixture of rosewater and sandalwood oil to "wash away" the sins of the year. Essential oil of sandalwood is derived from the wood of the sandalwood tree, via steam distillation.

MEDICINAL

Sandalwood oil is probably best known as an ingredient of perfumes and scented cosmetics, either as an essence in its own right, as a complementary fragrance in most rose types, or as a fixative. It also has preservative qualities which help to give creams and lotions a longer life. The oil is an excellent facial oil, being particularly soothing and emollient for dry, or irritated and sensitive skin, as it helps cleanse, heal, and soften. Sandalwood oil has a potent calming effect on the nerves and digestive system, making it very helpful for an upset stomach. The rich, woody aroma provides a relaxing and supportive environment for meditation, and promotes confidence and well-being. If you are feeling cold, a few drops of sandalwood oil in a hot bath will leave you wonderfully warm.

PROPERTIES

Digestive • calming • relaxing • soothing • softening and healing for skin • antispasmodic • antidepressant • sedative • warming

Sandalwood

Santalum album

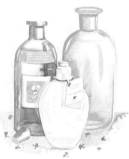

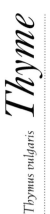

Thyme

Thymus vulgaris

DESCRIPTION AND HISTORY

*R*udyard Kipling described the scent of thyme as being "like the dawn in Paradise". It is a quintessential "summer herb", producing a stronger fragrance in hot sun, the aromatic oil being drawn out by the heat. Essential oil of thyme is obtained from the flowering tops of the plant via steam distillation.

MEDICINAL

Thyme was commonly mentioned in early medical texts as an antiseptic, a decongestant, a respiratory treatment, and a digestive aid. Natural therapists still use oil of thyme in the same manner. The Romans too used thyme for digestion and as a remedy for "melancholy" — or hangovers. It is also said to retard hair loss. Diluted in distilled water, thyme oil is a good general tonic and assists the circulatory and immune systems. In vapourization it fights infection. The oil is strengthening mentally and emotionally as well as physically.

PROPERTIES

Antiseptic • disinfectant • circulatory • stimulating • respiratory • nervine • cleansing and toning for skin • muscle relaxant

CAUTION

Avoid use during pregnancy.

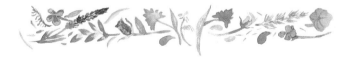

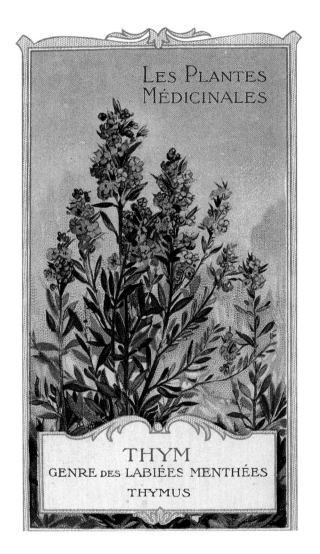

LES PLANTES
MÉDICINALES

THYM
GENRE DES LABIÉES MENTHÉES

THYMUS

PICTURE CREDITS

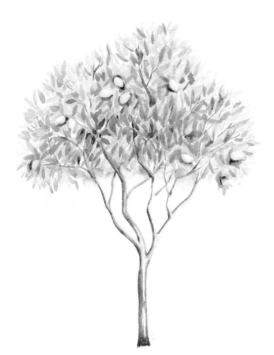

Illustrated by Sue Ninham

Designed by Catherine Martin
Set in Weiss on Quark Xpress
Printed in Singapore by Tien Wah Pte Ltd

Published by Lansdowne Publishing Pty Ltd
Level 5, 70 George Street, Sydney, NSW 2000

This 1994 edition published by Crescent Books, distributed by
Random House Value Publishing, Inc.,
40 Engelhard Avenue, Avenel, New Jersey 07001

Random House
New York • Toronto • London • Sydney • Auckland

Managing Director: Jane Curry
Production Manager: Sally Stokes
Publishing Manager: Deborah Nixon
Project editor: Kirsten Tilgals

First published in 1994

Reprinted 1995

ISBN 0-517-12067-4

A CIP catalog record for this book is available from the Library of Congress.

NOTE FROM PUBLISHER
The author, publisher and distributor cannot accept any responsibility for misadventure
resulting from the use of essential oils or any other therapeutic methods that are
mentioned in this book.